Tidi Talks:
PERIODS

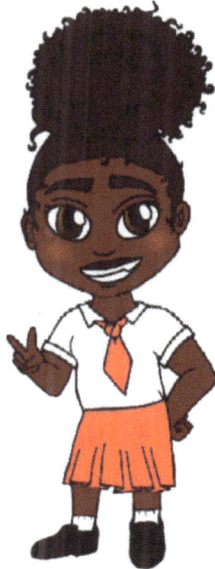

Farah C. Fortune
Dr Nokukhanya Khanyile
Thandzile Ndlovu

THANK YOU

One of the greatest gifts my mother ever gave me was knowledge about my body. I hope this book will give that gift to many parents and their children. Thank you to my parents Zanele and Bongani Ndlovu for all they have done for me. My sister Simnikiwe Ndlovu, who never misses a chance to remind me the joy a book can bring. My friends, who remind me daily of my capabilities. To my daughter, Zimasa Ndlovu. This is so you can see a book with faces like yours and names as powerful as yours. I carry you in every breath I take Sana Lwam!

Thandzile Ndlovu

To the girl I am learning from, the girl I am, to my beautiful revelation - Liepollo- and all the girls that will come, I pray that you use this book to help improve your mental health as well as uplifting the girls you are going to meet.

Dr Nokukhanya Khanyile

To my daughter, Laila, who has allowed me to blossom into the woman I am today, for her. My mother, the woman who moulded me & my family that celebrate the woman I am still becoming. To all the women & girls that gain from this book, thank you for letting us teach you & thank you Thandazile & Nokukhanya for believing in me.

Farah C. Fortune

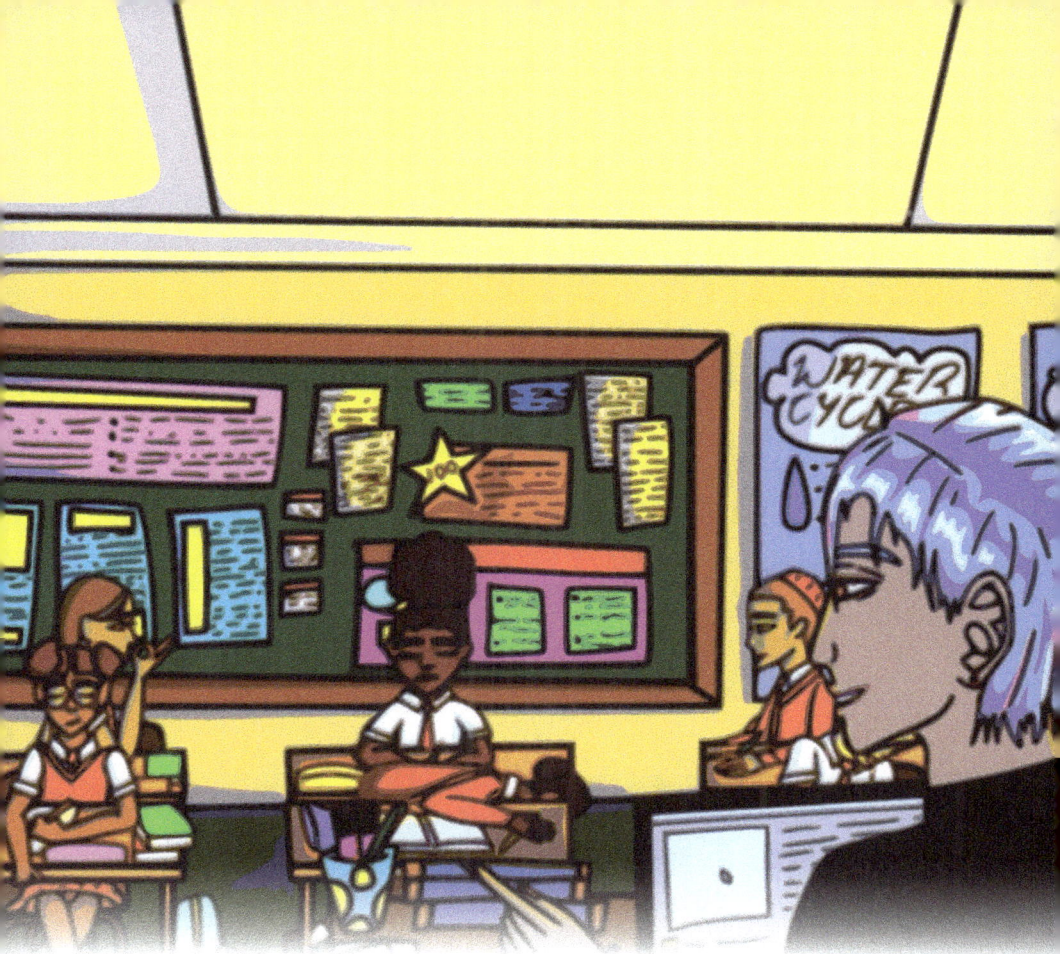

It was the last lesson of the day and all the kids in Teacher Terry's class were finishing off their class activities. "Boys and girls! Please don't forget that tomorrow Sister Zimasa from the local clinic will be coming to talk to us about periods. As always, I expect you to bring your best manners and be on your best behaviour," she said.

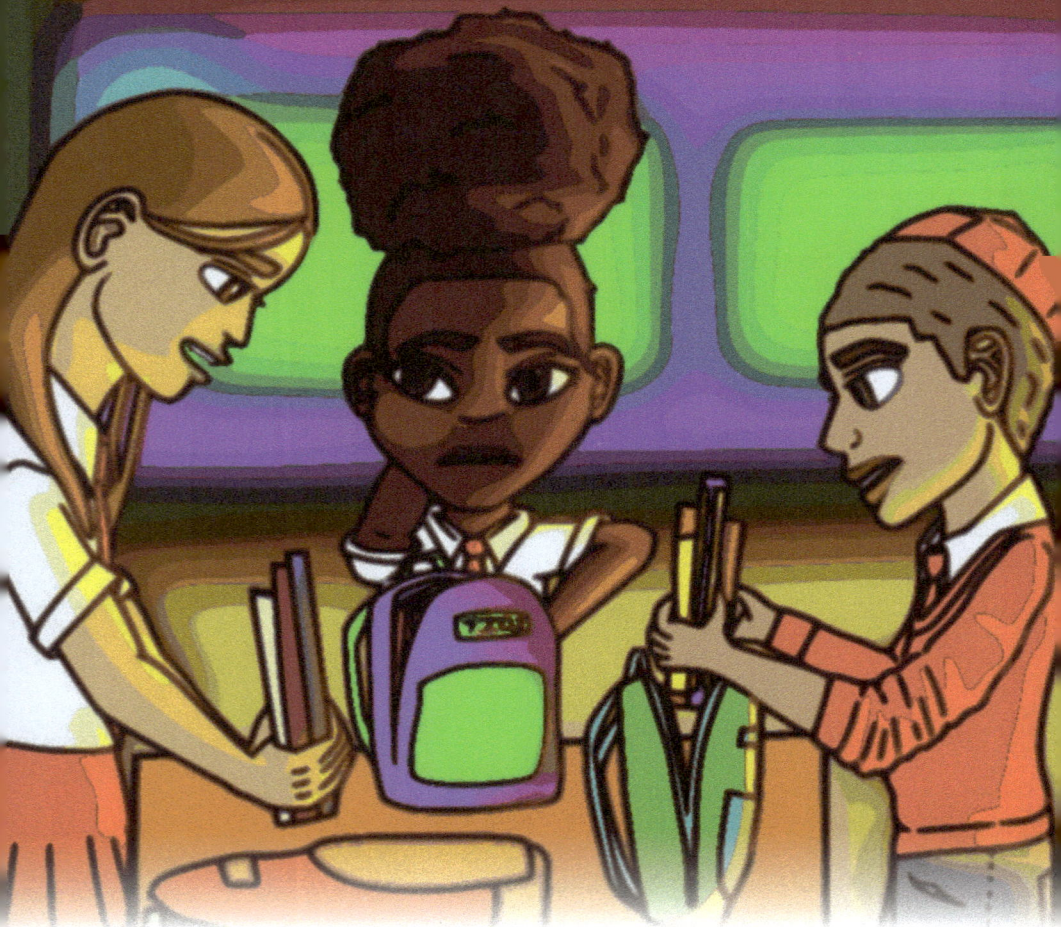

"I forgot all about that talk!" Tidimalo said to Taariq and Laila. "I just want to know why I need to be there? I won't ever get a period." said Taariq, annoyed. "Well, I don't want my crush to hear about how soon I'm going to start bleeding everywhere!" sighed Laila. Tidimalo asked, "Bleeding everywhere? Why would that happen?"

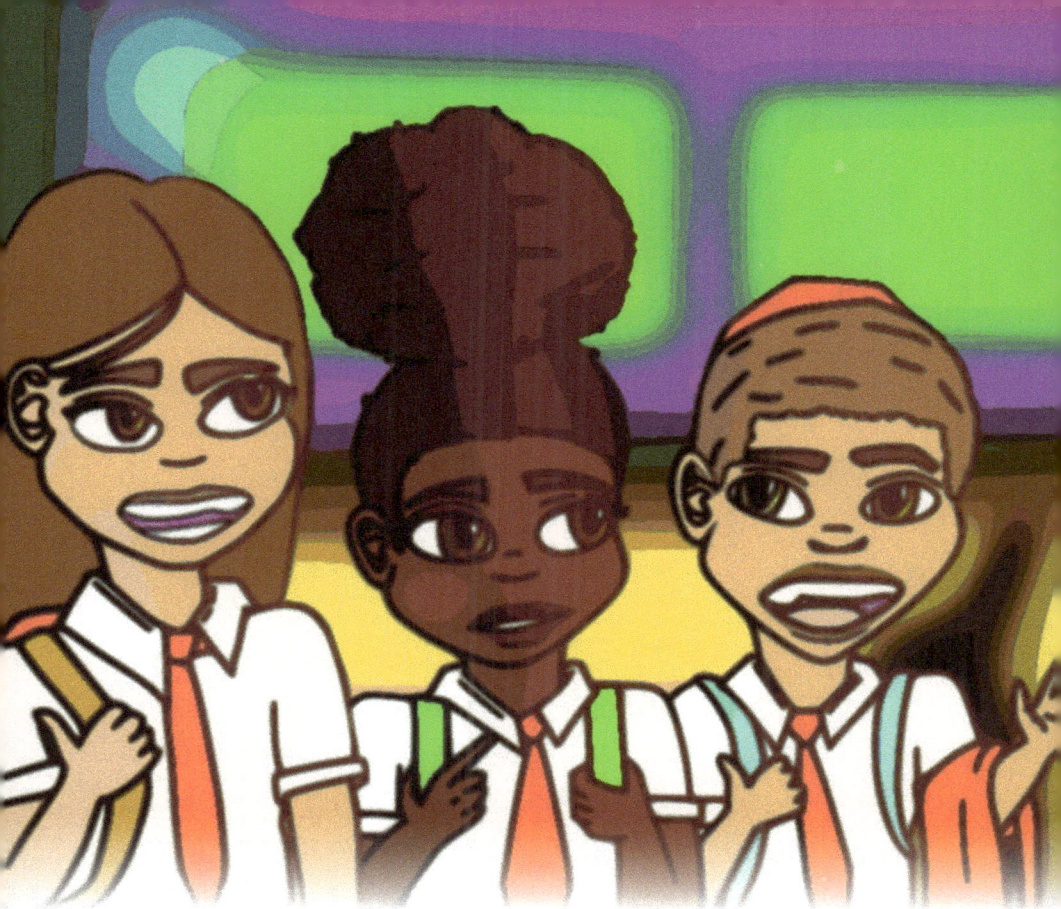

"Yeah, I don't think that's how it works Laila?" laughed Taariq. "How would you know Taariq? Like you said, you won't bleed!" replied Laila. "I know, but I have sisters and I've never seen them bleed everywhere. All I know is that they get really mean sometimes and my mom says it's because of their period." As Taariq finished his sentence, the bell rang for the end of the day.

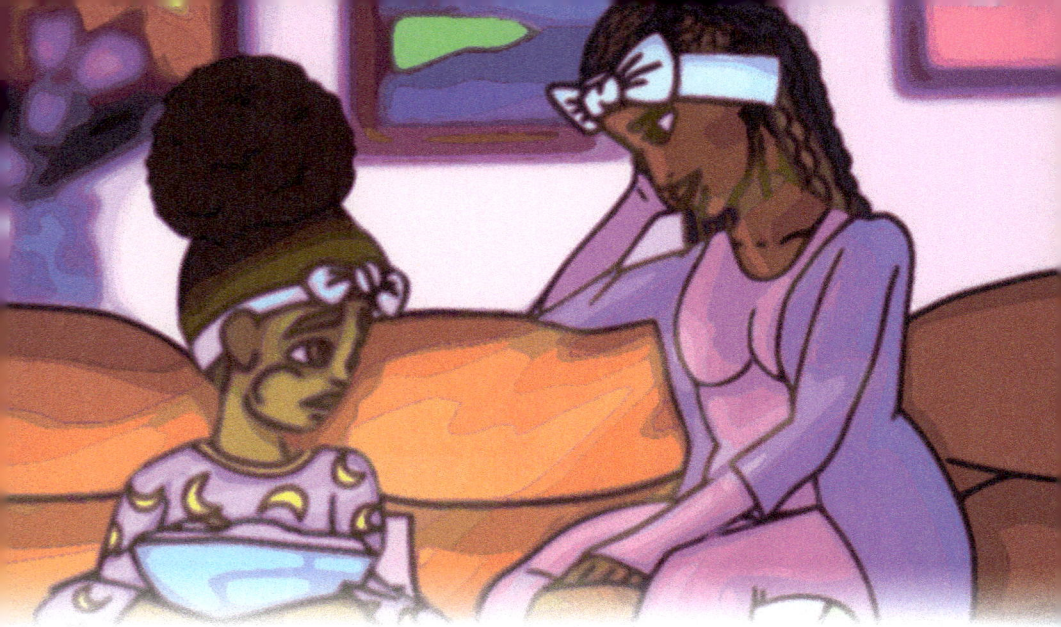

Later that night, Tidimalo and Mama were watching TV quietly when Tidimalo remembered the talk happening at school the next day. She turned to Mama and asked, "Mama, what's a period?" A little surprised Mama replied, "Where did you hear about periods, Tidimalo?" Jumping up excitedly, Tidimalo told Mama that Sister Zimasa was coming to school the next day to tell her class all about periods. Mama told Tidimalo to sit down next to her. "Tidi, periods are something everyone with a womb gets. A womb is something you have if you're born a girl. You can get your period from around the age of 9 years old," Mama said.

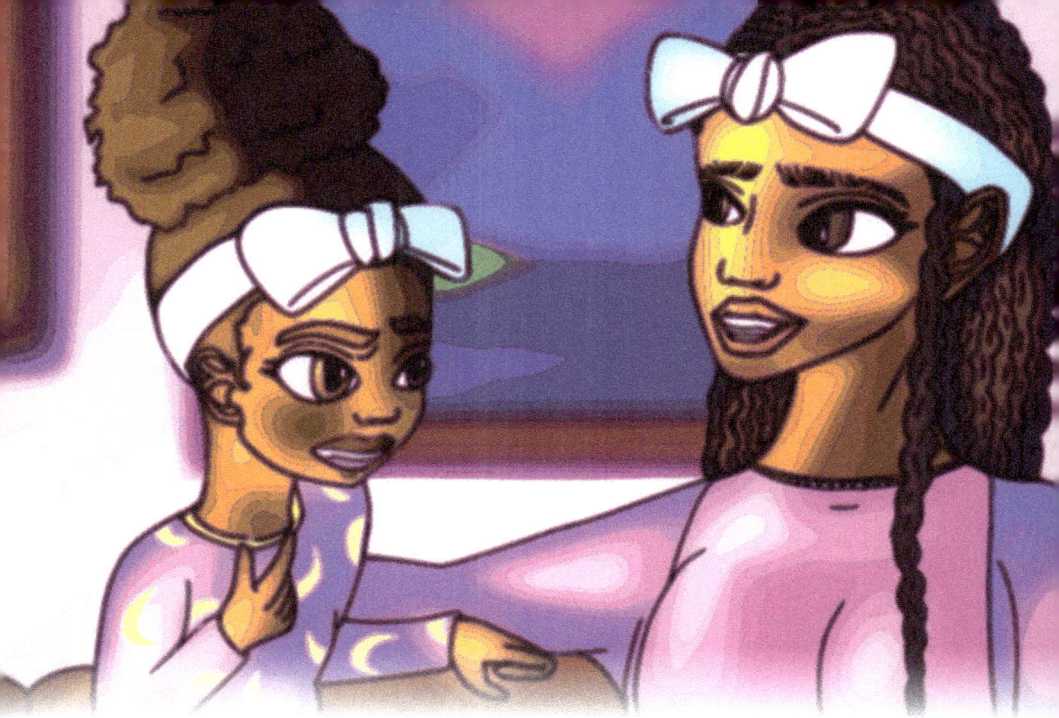

"So, I can get my period anytime now," Tidi said a little worried. Mama noticed how scared she looked and quickly said, "Don't be scared Tidi. There's nothing to worry about." Tidi's mind started spinning and she started firing questions at Mama. "So, what happens when you get your period Laila says blood will just come out of you from between your legs and you can't stop it!" Mama burst out laughing! "Yes, there is blood that comes out of your vagina but don't worry, there are ways to make the process a little easier. It will usually last between 3 to 7 days."

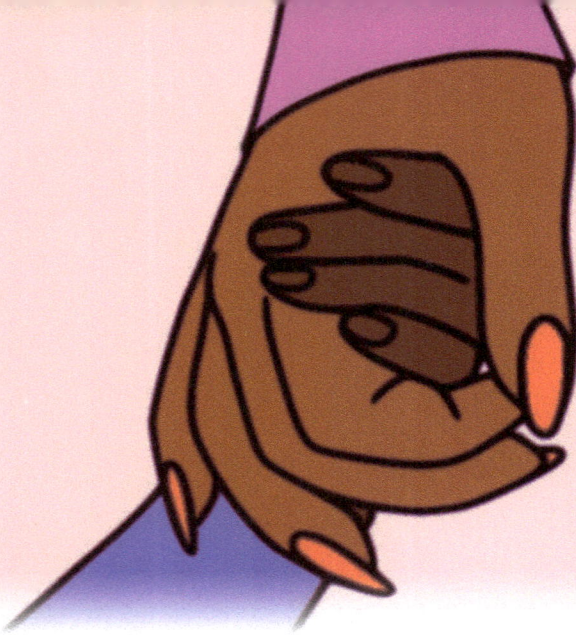

Tidi sat there for a second, thinking about what Mama had just told her and decided to ask more questions. "What's fertilized, Mama?" she asked. "Well," said Mama, "Why don't you save some of these questions for Sister Zimasa and we can chat some more when you get home tomorrow?" Tidi decided to write down her questions, but as she sat writing, Mama could see the worry on her face. Mama wanted to help her feel better. "A period generally happens every month and to make sure the blood doesn't mess on your clothes you can use a pad, a tampon, or a menstrual cup to catch the blood. Come with me I'll show you."

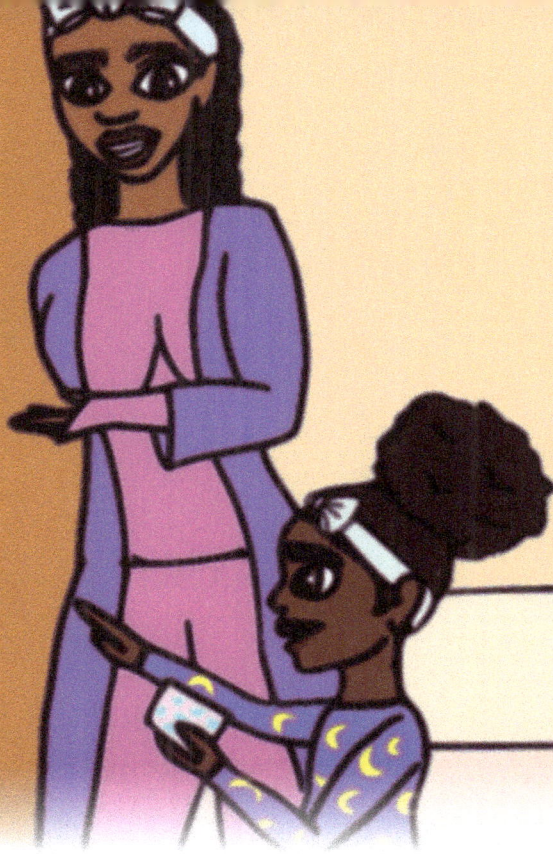

She took Tidimalo by the hand and walked to her wardrobe to show Tidi what they all look like. "A period is normal. Although, sometimes, when you get it, your body can feel a little weird. Don't let anyone make you feel it isn't okay. I'll put a pad in your bag to take to school with you just in case you need it." Tidimalo very excitedly said, "Thank you Mama! When Sister Zimasa speaks tomorrow, I'll know what she's talking about!"

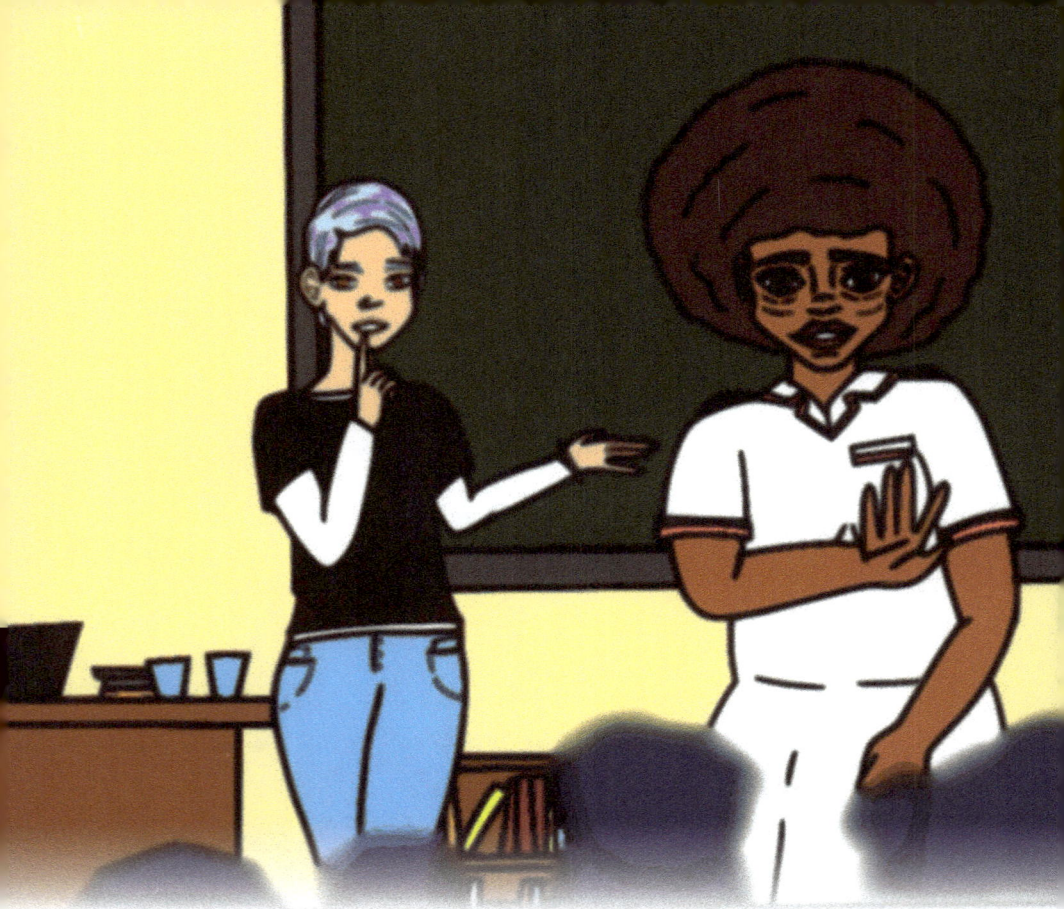

Tidimalo, Taariq and Laila walked into their class after break. When they sat down, they noticed Sister Zimasa in her nursing uniform in the class. Teacher Terry asked everyone to be quiet and introduced Sister Zimasa. "Everyone, I'd like you all to greet Sister Zimasa, who has come to give us an important health talk." The class responded, "Good morning, Sister Zimasa!"

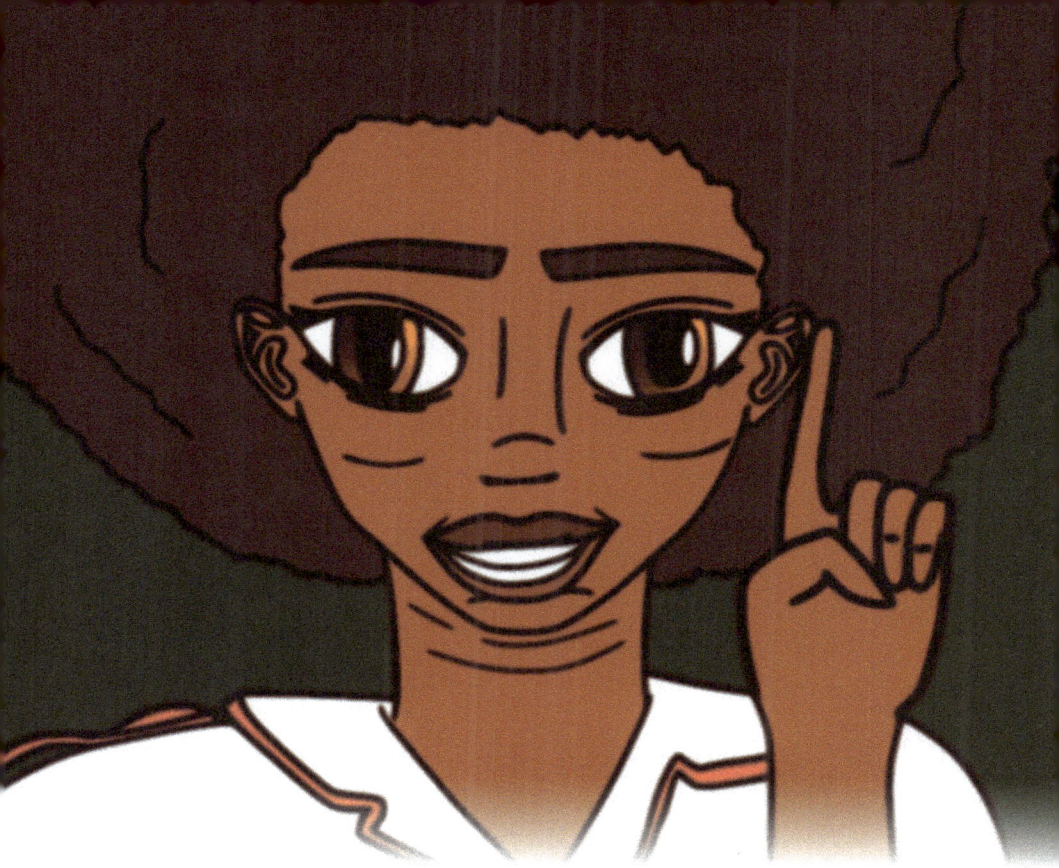

"Good morning class!" Sister Zimasa said. "I'm so excited to be here to speak to you about a very important topic: your period!" The students in the class all looked around at each other, some were confused, and others looked embarrassed. Tidimalo looked at Laila with an excited look on her face. She could get some important answers to the questions they had! "Can anyone tell me what a period is?" asked Sister Zimasa.

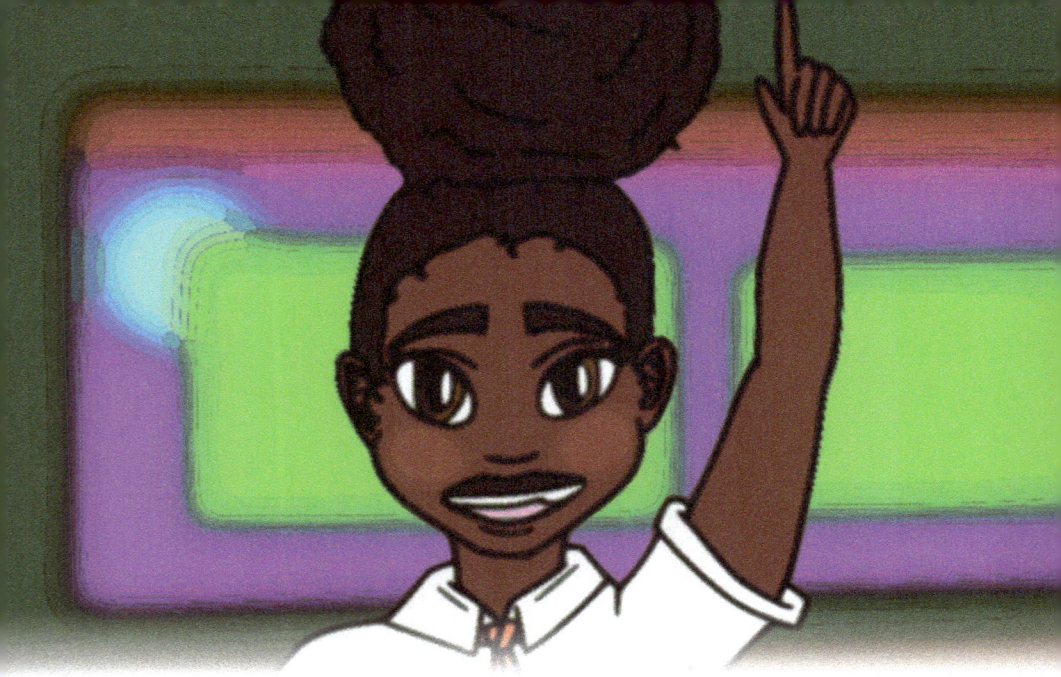

Tidimalo looked at her classmates and saw that nobody wanted to answer, so she put up her hand. "Yes?" Sister Zimasa said to her. "My mama says that a period is something that happens every month if you are a girl, where you have some blood coming out of your private parts, and you get weird feelings in your body." Sister Zimasa was happy with the answer that Tidimalo gave. "That's correct! You start to menstruate, or have your period, when your body goes through puberty," she started explaining. "Puberty is the process where your body goes from looking like a child to looking like a grown up."

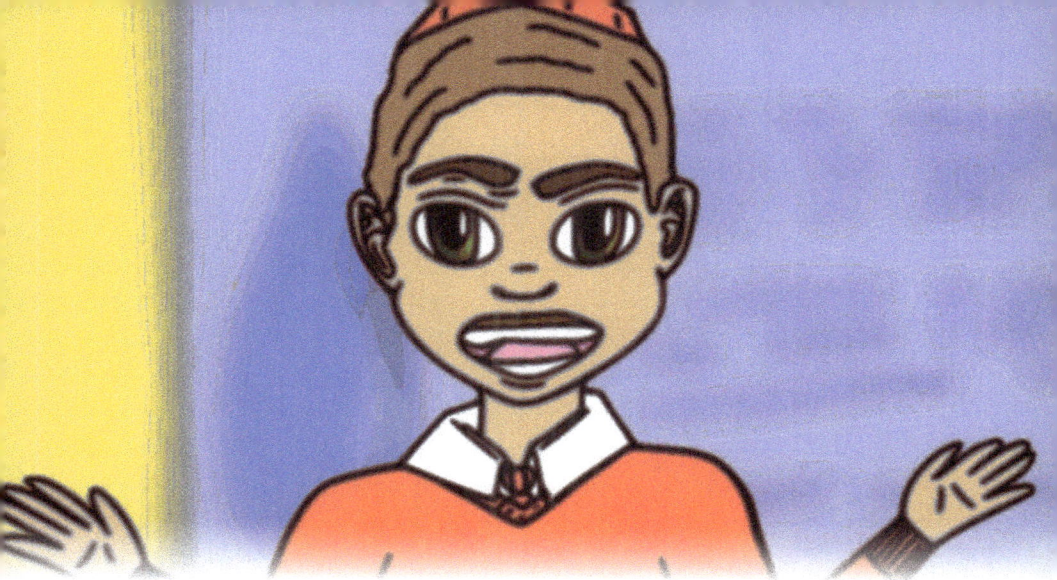

Taariq was terribly confused! He put his hand up and asked, "Does this mean I will also get my period? I also want to be a grown up!" Sister Zimasa smiled. "That's a very good question, Taariq! Only girls who have a vagina and a uterus, also called a womb, will have their period. Other signs of puberty include hair under your arms or over your vagina, a watery substance coming from the vagina or growng breasts." Taariq was still confused. "So how do boys become grown-ups", he asked. "They also get hair that grows under their arms, over their penis, on their face and on their body. They get a deeper voice, and they start to grow taller," Sister Zimasa explained.

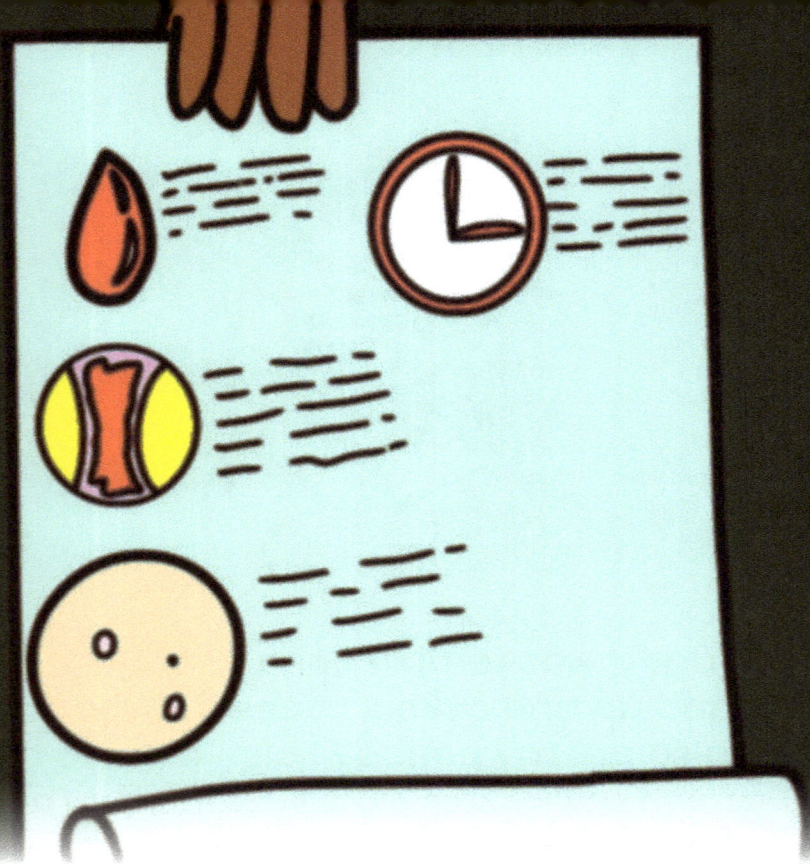

Sister Zimasa then went to her bag and pulled out a poster that had some important information about periods on it. She started explaining, "Your period can start anytime between the ages of 9 and 16 years old. Because every girl is different, you can all start at different ages." Tidi looked around the room and wondered who was on their period. She got a little bit worried because she was not sure when her time would come.

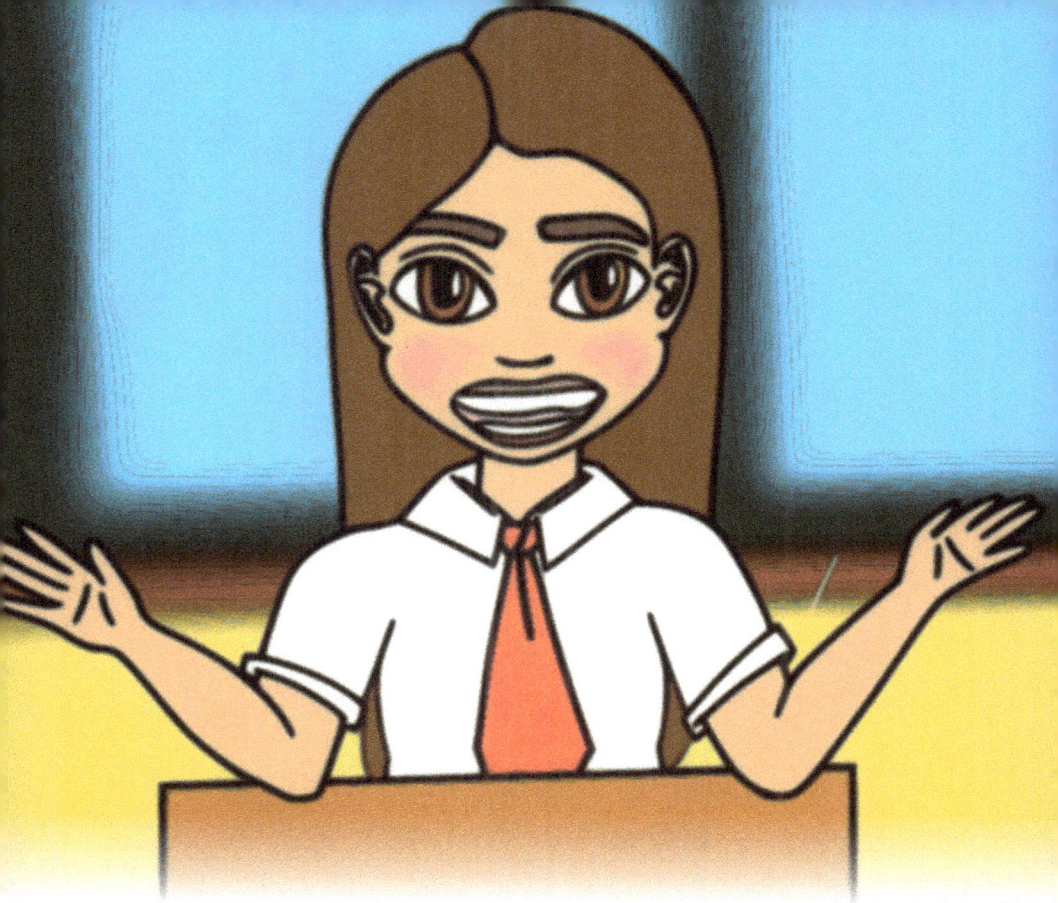

Laila put up her hand to ask a question, "Sister Zimasa, how will I know when my period is going to come?" Sister Zimasa answered, "That's a very good question! We can't say the exact date, but there are some signs that you can look out for. Your breasts will start to get bigger; hair will grow under your arms or between your legs, or you will see a sticky watery substance on your panty."

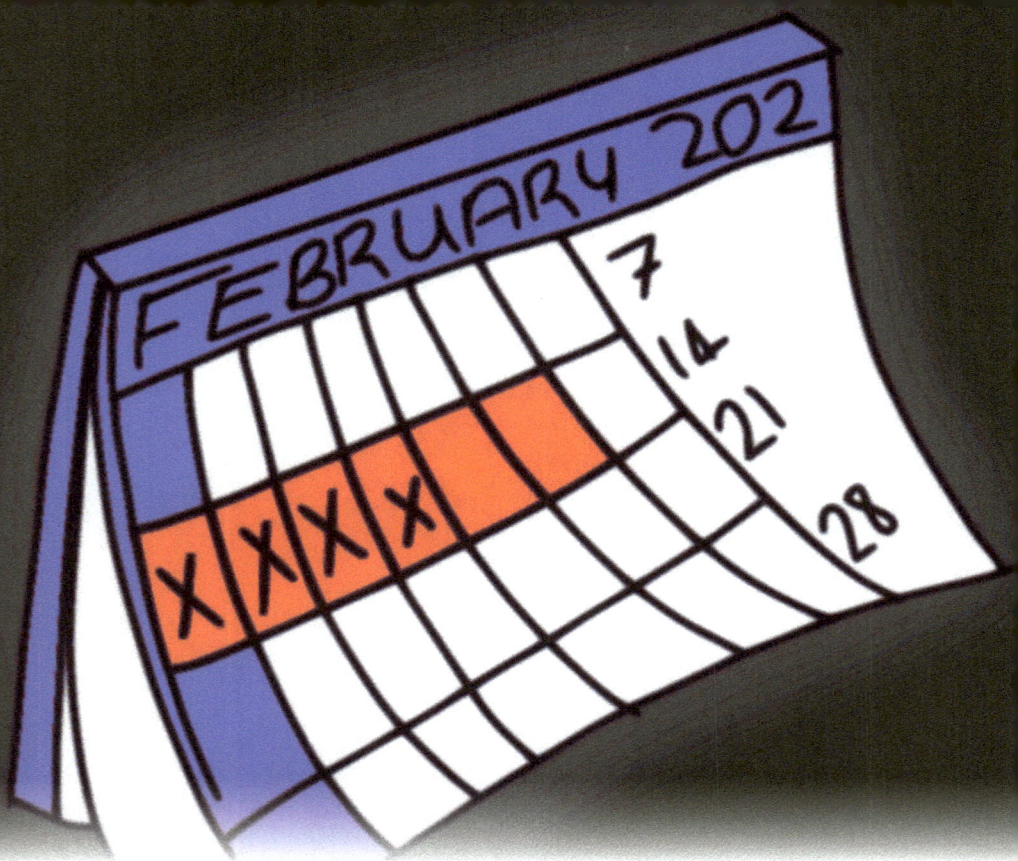

All of the boys in the class said, "Ewwwww!" But Sister Zimasa gently told them that it's completely normal. She then explained that when this happens, you can wear a panty liner. Sister Zimasa carried on explaining, "Usually, a girl's period will come every 21 to 35 days. If you mark it on a calendar, it will be easier to track, and you'll be able to prepare yourself better, and overtime understand the signals your body is sending you."

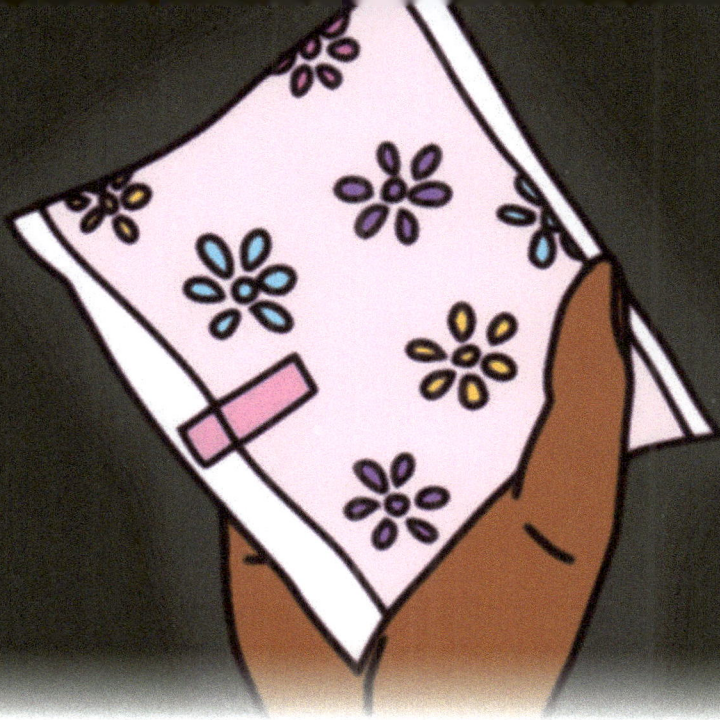

At this point, she reached into her bag and pulled out a VERY big packet. "I've seen that before!" said one of the girls in the class. "My mommy uses that! Is that a panty liner?" Sister Zimasa smiled and pulled out one of the pads from the packet. "This is a pad. You wear it on your panty during your period to catch the fluids that come out of your vagina. Not only blood comes out, but a watery fluid." Laila's eyes went wide. She put up her hand. "If I'm bleeding, does that mean I'm going to die?" Everyone looked at Sister Zimasa with worried faces.

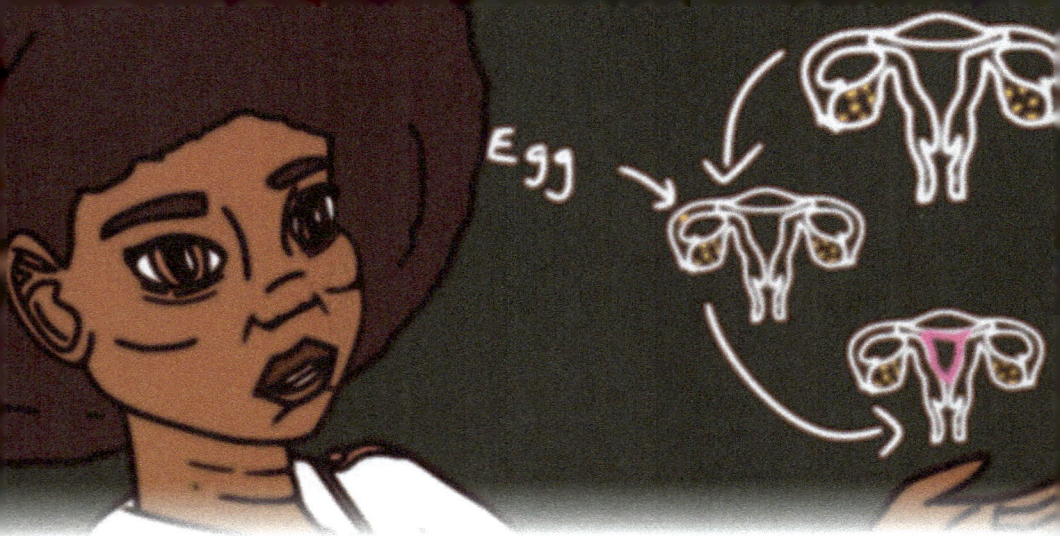

"You won't die Laila. Only about a teaspoon of blood comes out from the first day of your period until the end. You will need to wear pads for about 3 to 7 days." Everyone let out a big sigh of relief! Sister Zimasa then explained that a period happens because it means that your reproductive cycle, the thing that means you can make a baby, has begun working. Everyone looked around, and Teacher Terry could see that the children were quite confused. She asked Sister Zimasa to explain what that was. "It's when someone is ready to have a baby and an egg in a woman's ovary needs to meet with sperm. Sperm comes from a man. To fertilize, the egg and sperm must meet. This is how babies are made."

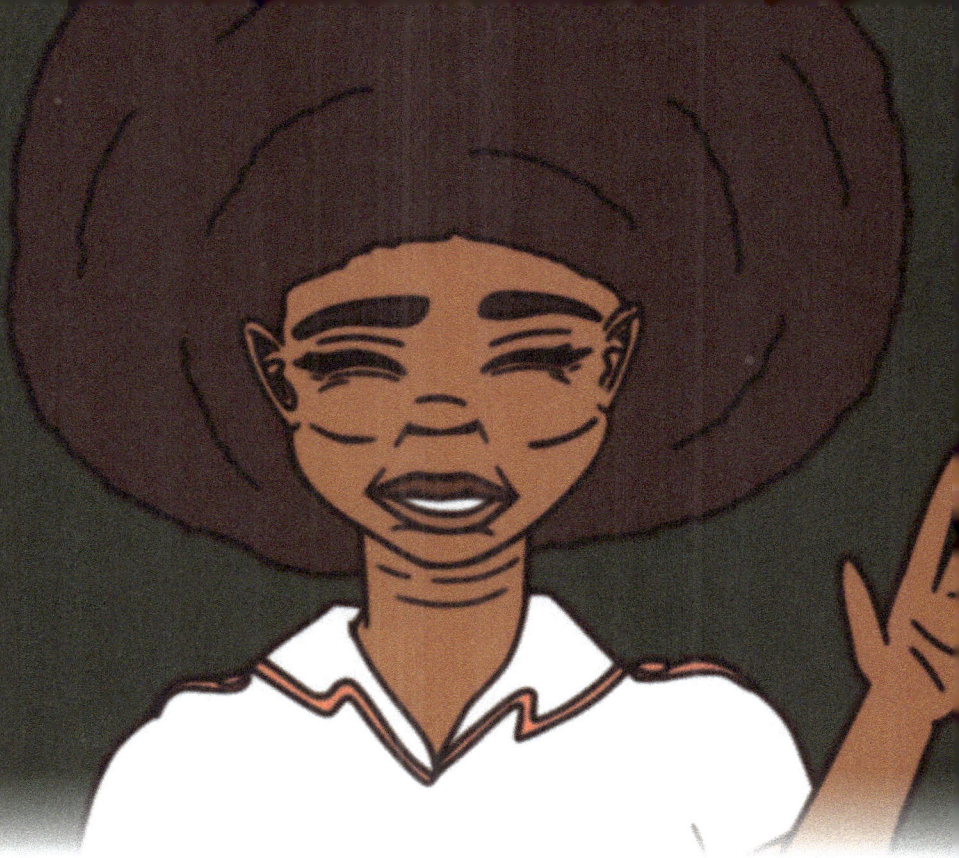

Teacher Terry was so happy that everyone was asking so many questions, but saw that the bell was about to ring for the end of the class. She apologised for having to stop the lesson and thanked Sister Zimasa for coming to teach the class about periods. "If anyone has any more questions, you can come and visit me at the clinic. You can also ask Teacher Terry or your parents for some help getting there."

17

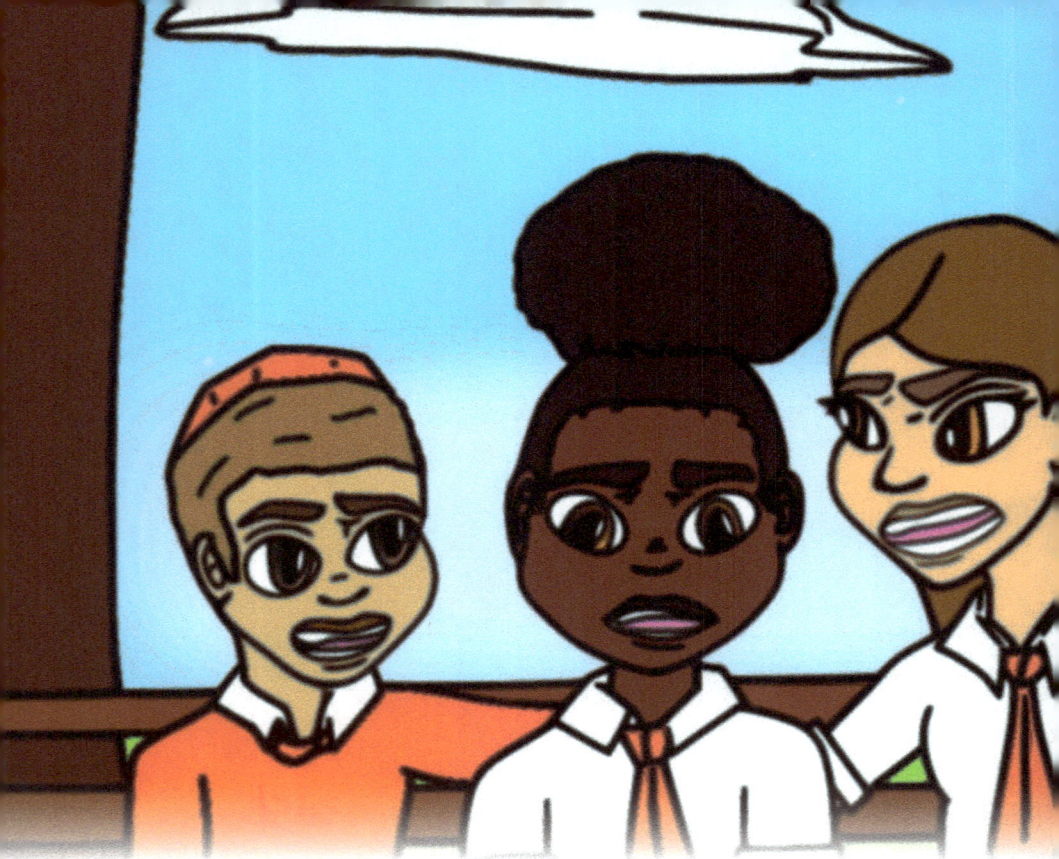

The following week Laila, Tidi and Taariq were chilling in their usual break time spot. Today something seemed off with Tidi; she was quieter and more reserved than usual. Laila asked, "Hey Tidi, what's wrong? You seem rather quiet today." Taariq added, "Yeah, you haven't made any funny jokes. What's going on?" Tidi answered, "I'm not sure, but I am feeling weird, my tummy hurts. I am going to get something to drink."

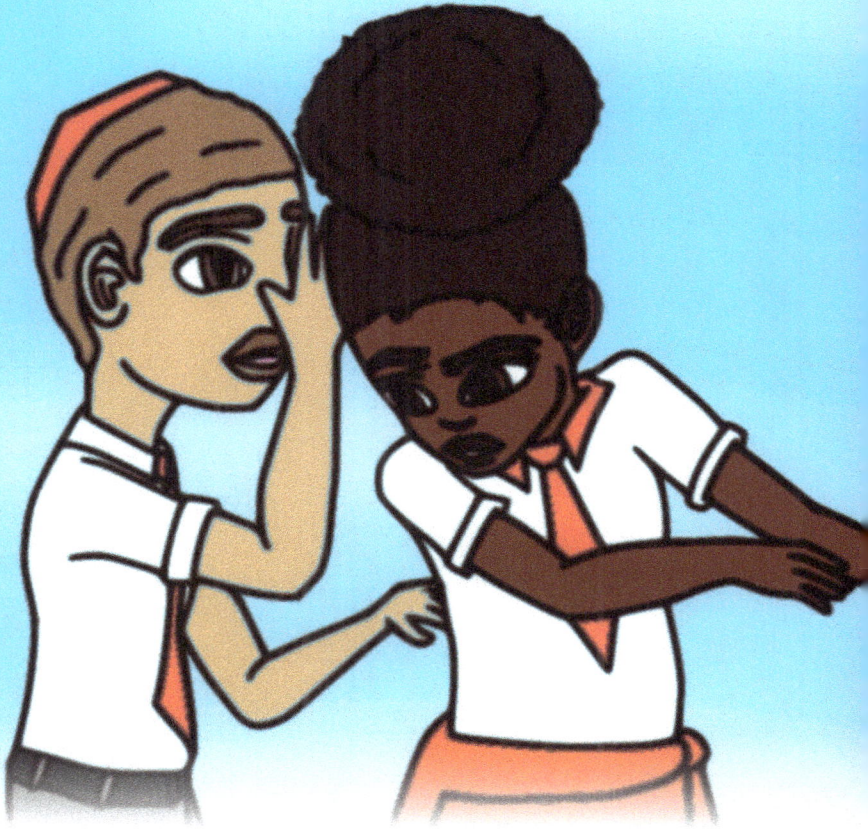

As Tidimalo stood up, Taariq noticed a red spot on the back of her skirt. He quickly got up, took off his jersey and wrapped it around her waist. He whispered in her ear, "I think you've started your period." Tidimalo gasped, "Oh goodness, I'm so glad I have a pad in my bag!" Laila, Tidimalo and Taariq walked to the bathroom. Laila went inside, while Taariq waited outside.

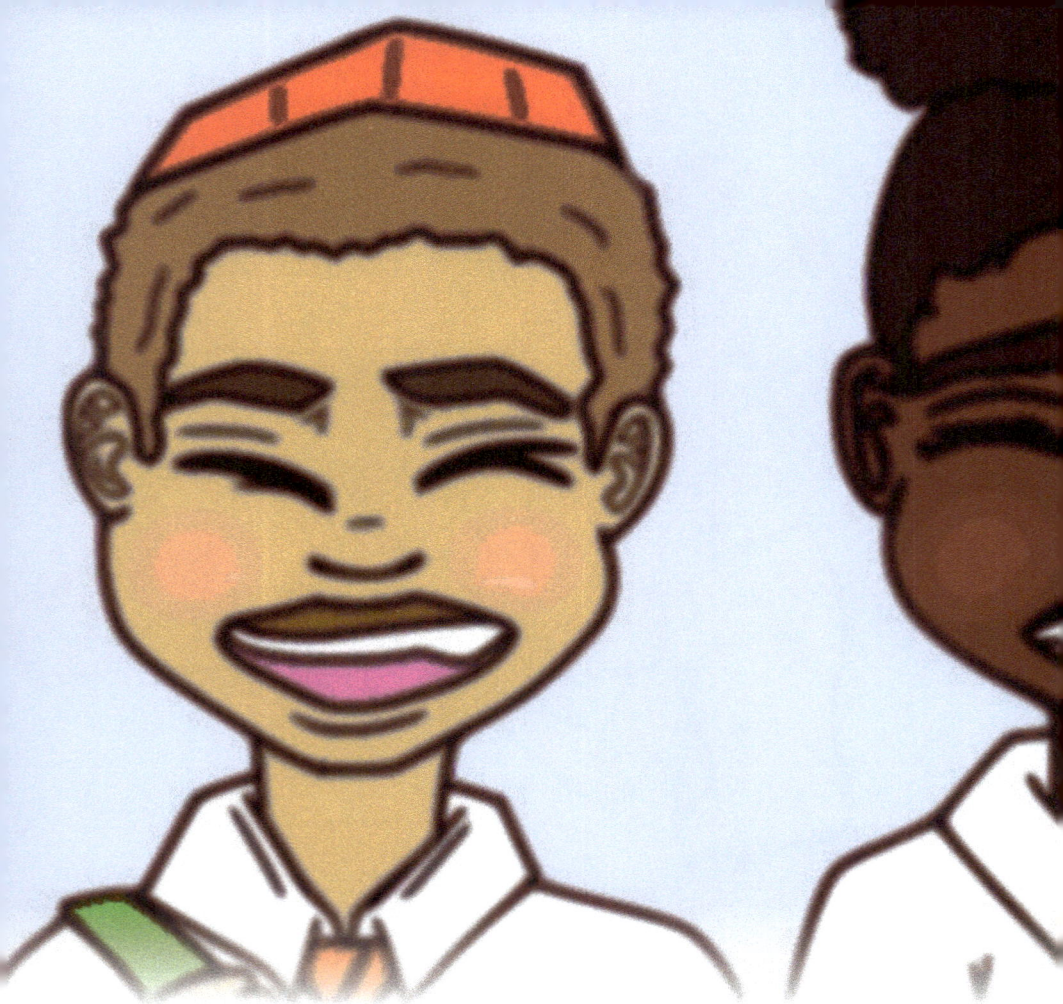

Laila asked Tidi if she knew how to put the pad on properly. She couldn't remember what Sister Zimasa taught them. Tidi answered, "Yes! I am super glad this is happening after that talk and the conversation with my mom. I feel more at ease because I know what to do." Tidi put on her pad and tried to clean up her skirt

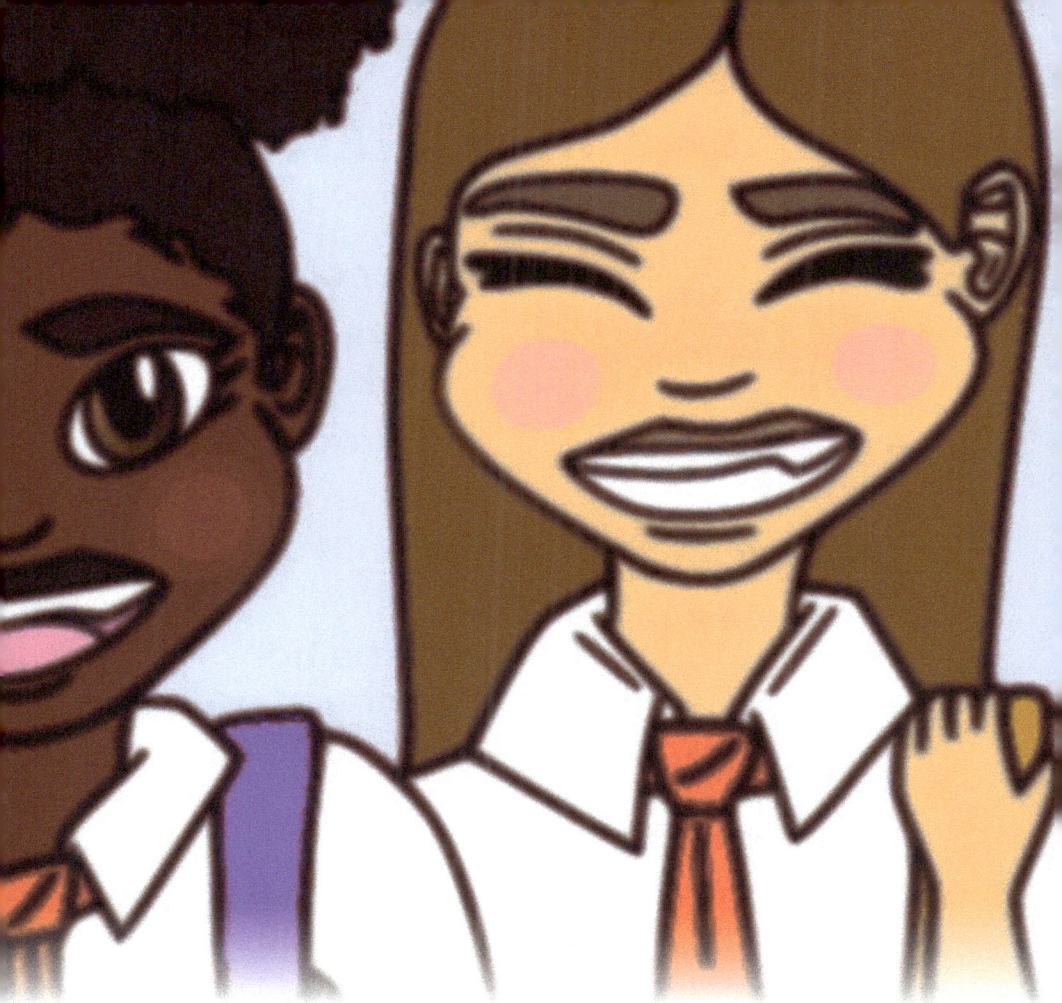

as much as she could before returning to break. Outside the bathroom, Taariq said he was feeling happy that they at least knew why Tidi wasn't feeling so great earlier, that attending the talk was helpful after all! Laila added, "That talk was helpful for all of us!" "Definitely!" Tidi agreed.

NOTES FOR PARENTS

Let's get started

- Show the children the cover of the book.
- Discuss what the characters are wearing and what they look like.
- Ask the children which character is their favourite and why.
- Read the title of the book with the children.
- Ask them what they think the book is about based on the information on the cover page.

Let's jump into it

- Read from page 1 up to page 6 to the children, while they follow as you read. Model reading with expression and taking note of punctuation.
- Ask the children how they think Tidi could make the process easier?
- Continue reading from page 7 up to page 10.
- Ask the children why they think Tidi's classmates did not want to answer Sister Zimasa's question?

Let's wrap it up

- Ask the children to read page 11 up to page 16 aloud to you.

- Recap the information Sister Zimasa shared with the class.

- Ask the children what information they wish Sister Zimasa had shared with the class.

- Ask the children what question they would ask Sister Zimasa if she visited their school.

- Ask the children to read the last few pages of the book.

- Ask the children who their favourite character in the book was and why.

USEFUL CONTACTS

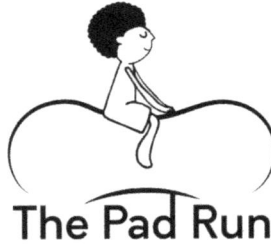

The Pad Run

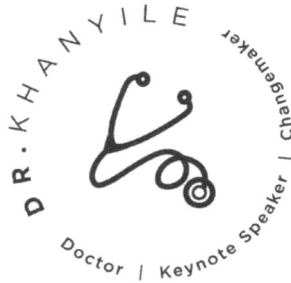

Tidi Talks: @tiditalksseries

Farah Fortune: @fcfortune

Dr Nokukhanya Khanyile: @dr_khanyile

Thandazile Ndlovu: @teacherthandi

The Pad Run: @thepadrun

Email: info@thepadrun.com or
tiditalksseries@gmail.com